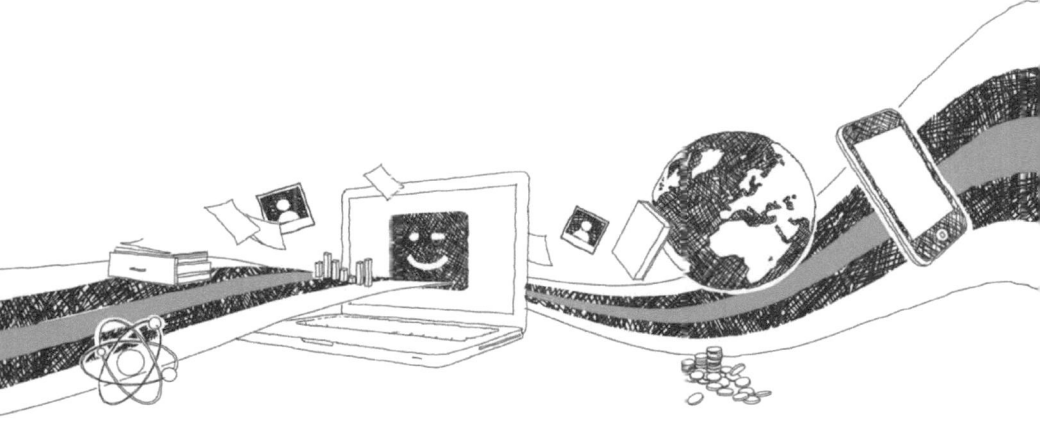
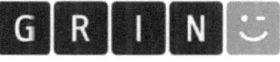

Badria Munir

Career Trends in Female Medical Students. A study at Allama Iqbal Medical College / Jinnah Hospital, Lahore

GRIN Publishing

Bibliographic information published by the German National Library:

The German National Library lists this publication in the National Bibliography; detailed bibliographic data are available on the Internet at http://dnb.dnb.de .

Imprint:

Copyright © 2014 GRIN Verlag GmbH
Print and binding: Books on Demand GmbH, Norderstedt Germany
ISBN: 978-3-656-87624-3

This book at GRIN:

http://www.grin.com/en/e-book/286633/career-trends-in-female-medical-students-a-study-at-allama-iqbal-medical

GRIN - Your knowledge has value

Since its foundation in 1998, GRIN has specialized in publishing academic texts by students, college teachers and other academics as e-book and printed book. The website www.grin.com is an ideal platform for presenting term papers, final papers, scientific essays, dissertations and specialist books.

Visit us on the internet:

http://www.grin.com/

http://www.facebook.com/grincom

http://www.twitter.com/grin_com

"Career Trends in Female Medical Students"

STUDY CONDUCTED BY
NAME: BADRIA MUNIR

4TH YEAR MBBS
SESSION 2013-14

DEPARTMENT OF COMMUNITY MEDICINE
ALLAMA IQBAL MEDICAL COLLEGE

CARRIER TRENDS IN FEMALE MEDICAL STUDENTS

A study conducted at Allama Iqbal Medical College / Jinnah Hospital, Lahore.

By

BATCH D
4TH YEAR MBBS
SESSION 2013-14

DEPARTMENT OF COMMUNITY MEDICINE,
ALLAMAIQBAL MEDICAL COLLEGE, LAHORE

INDEX

List of Tables & Graphs

Abstract:

Background:

Choosing a specialty is a complex process and may be influenced by several factors. There were some changes in the career choices of medical students. Interest in some specialties like surgery, pediatrics, and obstetrics & gynecology declined.

Objective:

The objective of research is to evaluate career choices among female medical students.

Material and Methods:

Study Design:

Cross sectional Study

Study Setting and duration:

Study was done on students of Allama Iqbal Medical College,Lahore in the duration of three months.

Inclusion criteria:

Female Students of MBBS.

Data Collection and analysis:

A questionnaire was given; which was filled under supervision to female students of First year and 4th year.Analysis was done on SPSS version 17.

.Results:

About 87% of our respondents state that medicine is a well suited profession for girls, and out of these respondents 90% are willing to continue their profession after graduation. While 63% had the opinion that Gender will have potent influence over their choice of specialty in future More than 50% of respondents claimed that their

5

choice of specialty had changed owing to the amount of time they spent in this field and observed closely.

Conclusions:

Most of female medical undergraduate are satisfied with their career choice as being doctor. Families had strong influence of their choice of specialty.

Key words: Career choice, Gender, Medical under graduates

INTRODUCTION:

Purpose of the study is to investigate the Career choices among medical students. The area that is to explore in this research will be helpful for the students to determine the effects of selection, educational background, age and gender on strength of motivation to attend and pursue medical school.

Career is a person's "course or progress through life (or a distinct portion of life)". It is related to an occupation or a profession that usually involves special training or formal education,[1] and is considered to be a person's lifework.

Medicine is the field of applied science related to the art of healing by diagnosis, treatment, and prevention of disease.[2] It encompasses a variety of health care practices evolved to maintain and restore health by the prevention and treatment of illness in human beings.

Choosing a specialty is a complex process and may be influenced by several factors. There were some changes in the career choices of medical students. Interest in some specialties like surgery, pediatrics, and obstetrics & gynecology declined. But the popularity of controllable lifestyle fields such as radiology, psychiatry, dermatology, and ophthalmology has been increased. Controllable lifestyle specialties have been defined as those that allow more personal time free for rest, leisure, and family. With the increase of women into medicine has come the concern that women are responsible for a growing interest in medical specialties with controllable lifestyles and decreased interest in primary care specialties. Despite the increasing representation of women in medicine, little has been known about how gender has affected specialty choice.[4]

Career choice has generally been believed to be influenced by many factors including income, intellectual stimulation, role models, and prestige. Both men and women have been shown to select specialties based on some common factors like individual aptitude, personality, and positive clerkship experiences, while men place greater emphasis on prestige, income and manual dexterity skills than women. Although women have traditionally preferred specialties like pediatrics and obstetrics & gynecology, it has been supposed that the preferences of a specialty with a controllable lifestyle such as radiology, psychiatry, and rehabilitation medicine are more appealing to women who want to balance family and career responsibilities. If we do not change the system to encourage and enable women to contribute maximally to their profession, academic specialties can lose a major source of potential talent. The relatively stable work qualities of specialties in comparison with other medical disciplines would seem likely to appeal to female students or doctors.[4]

OBJECTIVES:

The objective of this study is to demonstrate career trends in female Medical students of first year and 4th year.

MATERIAL AND METHODS:

STUDY DESIGN:

- Cross sectional study

STUDY SETTING:

- Students of Allama Iqbal Medical College, Lahore

DURATION OF STUDY:

- Three months

SAMPLE SIZE: 345

SAMPLING TECHNIQUE:

- Non probability / purposive sampling

SAMPLE SELECTION:

Inclusion criteria: Female students of MBBS studying in Allama Iqbal Medical College,Lahore

Exclusion criteria: Students who were not regular in their curricular courses were excluded.

DATA COLLECTION PROCEDURE:

- A questionnaire was given to students who filled under supervision. It had 15 questions.

DATA ANALYSIS PROCEDURE:

Data entry and analysis was done on SPSS version 17. Mean and standard deviation was calculated for age ,father's occupation, mother's occupation and for every question stated in questionare.Analysis was done on SPSS 17.

RESULTS AND MAIN FINDINGS:

Table. 1 Age of Respondents

Statistics

Age

N	Valid	345
	Missing	0
Mean		20.0696
Median		20.0000
Mode		18.00
Std. Deviation		1.72560
Minimum		18.00
Maximum		24.00

Table. 1 Class of Respondents

Class

		Frequency	Percent	Valid Percent	Cumulative Percent
Valid	1st year	174	50.4	50.4	50.4
	2nd year	3	.9	.9	51.3
	3rd year	15	4.3	4.3	55.7
	4th year	153	44.3	44.3	100.0
	Total	345	100.0	100.0	

Graph 1.

Fathers Education

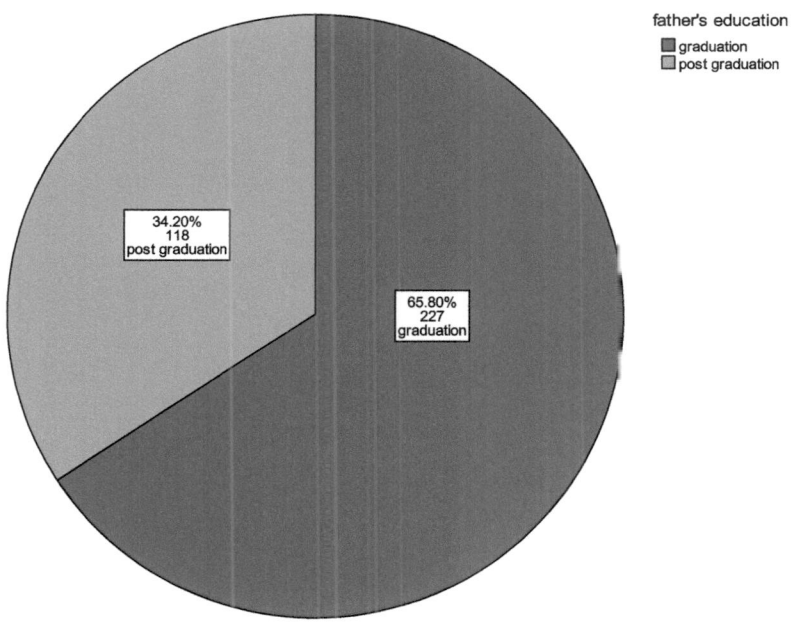

Graph 2.

Comparing Fathers Education

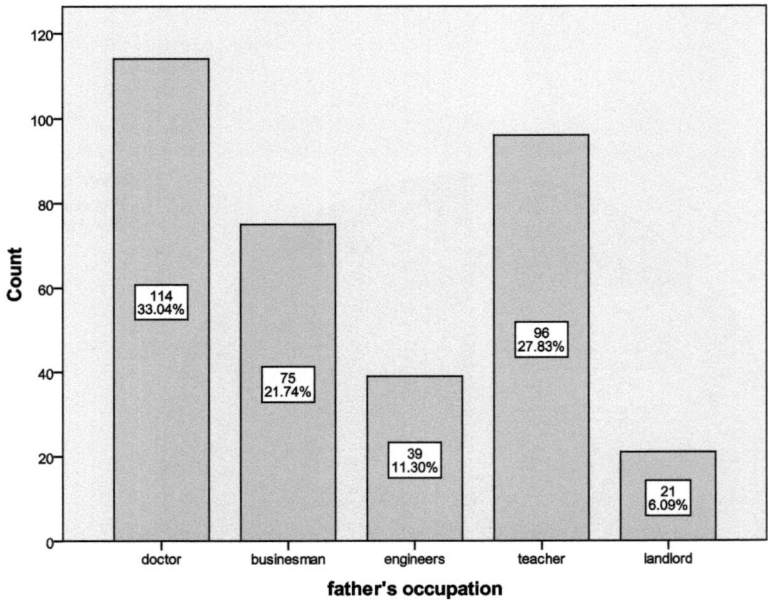

Graph 3.

Mother's Education:

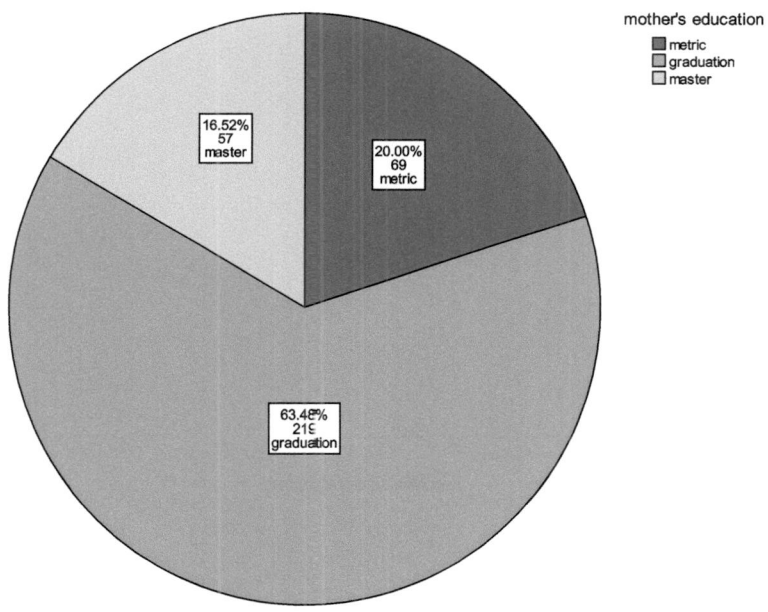

Mother's Occupation:

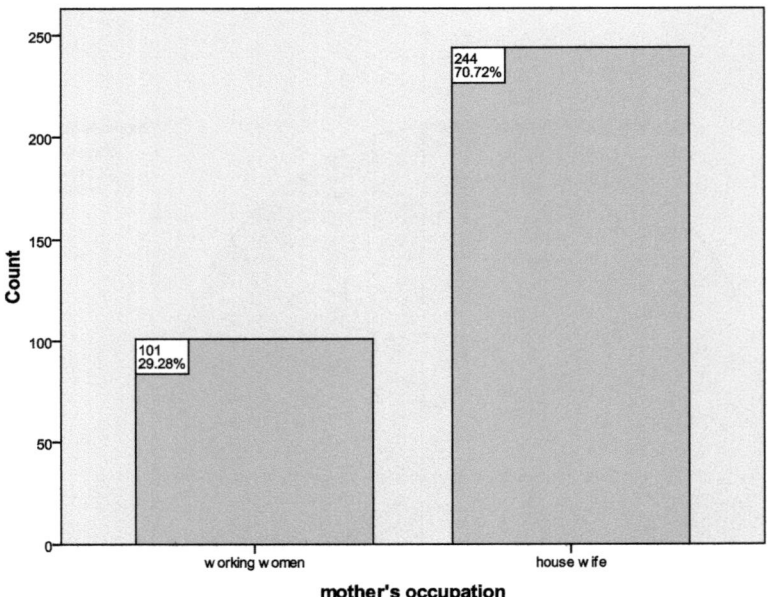

Graph 5.

Students Residence

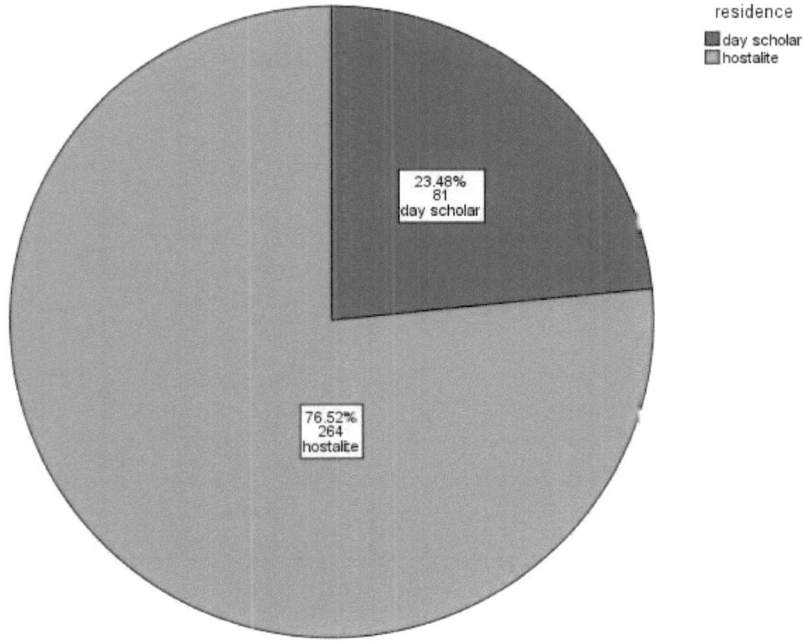

residence
- day scholar
- hostalite

23.48%
81
day scholar

76.52%
264
hostalite

Table 2.

Questionnaire and relative frequencies

$Trends Medical education (yes) Frequencies

	Responses		Percent of Cases
	N	Percent	
Is medical Profession best suited for girls in our country?	300	14.9%	87.0%
Are you planning to pursue your career after graduation?	319	15.9%	92.5%
Are you planning to do specialty in a particular field?	303	15.1%	87.8%
Do you think gender has some influence on your choice of specialization?	222	11.0%	64.3%
Do you think attitude of seniors would have any influence on your career?	198	9.8%	57.4%
Is there any change in your field of specialty over period of time you spent in Medical school?	183	9.1%	53.0%
Does your choice of specialization influenced by your current economical status?	84	4.2%	24.3%
In your opinion are physicians adequately compensated for they care they render?	105	5.2%	30.4%
Is there any bright career for female doctors in Surgery?	195	9.7%	56.5%
Do you think Gynae/Obs are the ultimate fields for female doctors?	102	5.1%	29.6%
Total	2011	100.0%	582.9%

a. Dichotomy group tabulated at value 1.

Table 3.

Reasons for choosing medical profession?

		Frequency	Percent	Valid Percent	Cumulative Percent
Valid	your own wish	264	76.5	76.5	76.5
	economical security	15	4.3	4.3	80.9
	parents enforcement	48	13.9	13.9	94.8
	social factors	18	5.2	5.2	100.0
	Total	345	100.0	100.0	

Table 4.

Main reason not choosing a Specialty?

	Frequency	Percent	Valid Percent	Cumulative Percent
Not planning to choosing specialty	42	12.2	12.2	12.2
I am looking for a specialty with good reputation and prestige	192	55.7	55.7	67.8
I want high income	47	13.6	13.6	81.4
lack of specialist in my country	34	9.9	9.9	91.3
I want to treat less complicated patients	30	8.7	8.7	100.0
Total	345	100.0	100.0	

17

Table 5.

Reason for not choosing particular specialty selection?

		Frequency	Percent	Valid Percent	Cumulative Percent
Valid	Own choice	321	93.0	93.0	93.0
	Family	18	5.2	5.2	98.3
	Friends	3	.9	.9	99.1
	practicing doctors	3	.9	.9	100.0
	Total	345	100.0	100.0	

Table 6.

Influnce of family

How much influence would your family have on your career?

		Frequency	Percent	Valid Percent	Cumulative Percent
Valid	no influence at all	36	10.4	10.4	10.4
	minor influence	36	10.4	10.4	20.9
	some influence	117	33.9	33.9	54.8
	strong influence	156	45.2	45.2	100.0
	Total	345	100.0	100.0	

RESULTS:

Age of Respondents: (table 1)

Mean age calculated for the girls studing in Medical field at the time was 20 yrs.Maximum Age was 24 and minimum was 18 yrs. SD calculated 1.75.Which concludes the fact that around 20 yrs is the age that female students usually come across the course of Medicine.(

Class Statistic (table 2)

174 students from 1st year and 153 students from 4th year were of particular interest.

Father's Education

65.80% female students had father's education Graduation or equivalent to Graduation. While 34.20% of fathers were Post Graduates.

Father's Occupation:

Our study on Father's occupation revealed that 33% of fathers of our respondents were Doctors,27 % were businessmen, 27.83% teachers and only 6% landlaord.This concludes that female students were influenced to some extent from Medical related person already present in their homes.

Mother's Education:

63% of respondents revealed that their mothers had education upto Graduation or equivalent to graduation.This indicated most of the educated families were inclined to get their daughters into some professional studies.

Questionnaire respond (table 2.)

About 87% of our respondants state that medicine is a well suited profession for girls,and out of these respondants 90% are willing to continue their profession after graduation.While 63% had the opinion that Gender will have potent influence over their choice of speciality in future. More than 50% of respondents claimed that their choice of speciality hhad changed owing to the amount of time they spent in this field and observed closely. In the current state of economics almost 30% of respondents stated that their speciality is not based on economic needs and also they are not satisfied with current economical wages of doctors. Regarding particular field of speciality 53% stated that surgery isn't fit for girls and GYNAE OBS is not ultimate end of female doctors.

Frequencies of reasons choosing the Medical Profession.(table 3.)

76% stated that it was their own choice.4.3% entered this profession for economical security.13% were enforced by parents.5.2% chose this profession for better social fact.

Main reason not choosing a Specialty?(table 4.)

12 stated that they don't want to choose any specialty after graduation.55% preffered to get into a field of good repute and prestige,13% wanted high income.9.9 % had the idea of serving the coutry in the fields which had deficient specialists .while 8.7 preffered their own comfort so as they will have to treat less complicated case.

Reason for not choosing particular specialty selection.(table 5)

93% said it was their own choice.5.2% said it was their family's choice.)0.9% friends and 0.9% practicing doctors.

Influence of family (table 6).

45% of girls came with the fact that their families had storng influence of their choice of specialty.while10.4 had minor or no influence at all.other 35% were under some influence.

DISCUSSON:

Over 60% of UK medical students are female, yet only 33% of applicants to surgical training are women. Role modelling, differing educational experiences and dis-identification in female medical students have been implicated in this disparity. We are yet to fully understand the mechanisms that link students' experiences with national trends in career choices. We employ a hitherto unused concept from the theory of communities of practice: paradigmatic trajectories. These are visible career paths provided by a community and are cited by Wenger as potentially the most influential factors shaping the learning of newcomers. Female students' experiences of surgery were strongly gendered; they were positioned as 'other' in the surgical domain. Four key processes--seeing, hearing, doing and imagining--facilitated the formation of paradigmatic trajectories, on which students could draw when making career decisions. Female students were unable to see or identify with other women in surgery. They heard about challenges to being a female surgeon, lacked experiences of participation, and struggled to imagine a future in which they would be successful surgeons. Thus, based on paradigmatic trajectories constructed from exposure to surgery, they self-selected out of surgical careers. By contrast, male students had experiences of 'hands-in' participation and were not marginalized by paradigmatic trajectories.[5]

The concept of the paradigmatic trajectory is a useful theoretical tool with which to understand how students' experiences shape career decisions. Paradigmatic trajectories within surgery deter female students from embarking on careers in surgery.

In our study 12 stated that they don't want to choose any specialty after graduation.55% preffered to get into a field of good repute and prestige,13% wanted high income.9.9 % had the idea of serving the country in the fields which had deficient specialists .while 8.7 preferred their own comfort so as they will have to treat less complicated case.93% said it was their own choice.5.2% said it was their family's choice.)0.9% friends and 0.9% practicing doctors. 45% of girls came with the fact that their families had strong influence of their choice of specialty.while10.4 had minor or no influence at all. Other 33% were under some influence. Another study done to characterize how female medical students perceive the role of gender within their medical education during the transition to the clinical curriculum. In 2006-2007, the authors conducted a qualitative study consisting of in-depth interviews with 12 third-year female medical students completing their first clinical clerkship. Participants were purposefully selected from a single New England medical school to represent a range of ages, ethnicities, and prior life experiences. And found that Participants (1) struggled to define their role on the wards and often defaulted to stereotypical gender roles, (2) perceived differences in the nature of their workplace relationships compared with the nature of male medical students' workplace relationships, (3) had gendered expectations of male and female physicians that shaped their interactions with clinical supervisors, (4) felt able to negotiate uncomfortable situations with patients but felt unable to negotiate uncomfortable situations with supervisors and attendings, and (5) encountered a "gender learning curve" on the wards that began to shape their self-view as future female physicians. [6]

In our study About 87% of our respondants state that medicine is a well suited profession for girls, and out of these respondents 90% are willing to continue their profession after graduation. While 63% had the opinion that Gender will have potent influence over their choice of speciality in future. More than 50% of respondents claimed that their choice of specialty had changed owing to the amount of time they spent in this field and observed closely. In the current state of economics almost 30% of respondents stated that their specialty is not based on economic needs and also they are not satisfied with current economical wages of doctors. Regarding particular field of specialty 53% stated that surgery isn't fit for girls and GYNAE OBS is not ultimate end of female doctors

The study concluded that despite increased numbers of women in medicine, issues of gender continue to have a substantial impact on the medical education of female students. Institutions can design interventions about gender issues in medicine that expand beyond a focus on sexual harassment to address the complex ways in which students are affected by issues of gender.

CONCLUSION:

Most of female medical undergraduate are satisfied with their career choice as being doctor. Families had strong influence of their choice of specialty.

REFERENCES:

1. Career (2014). The free Dictionary. Retrieved from http://www.thefreedictionary.com/career

2. Medicine (2014). Dictionary.com. Retrieved from http://dictionary.reference.com/browse/medicine

3. Theories of Career Choice (2005). Retrieved form https://www.kent.ac.uk/careers/Choosing/career-choice-theories.htm

4. Lee., C. L. (2012). Gender differences and specialty preference in medical career choice. Department of Pediatrics, Wonkwang University School of Medicine.

5. Hill E[1], Vaughan S. The only girl in the room: how paradigmatic trajectories deter female students from surgical careers. Med Educ. 2013 Jun;47(6):547-56. doi: 10.1111/medu.12134.

6. Babaria P[1], Abedin S, Nunez-Smith M. The effect of gender on the clinical clerkship experiences of female medical students: results from a qualitative study. Acad Med. 2009 Jul;84(7):859-66. doi: 10.1097/ACM.0b013e3181a8130c.